Unleash the Body Within

Real World Advice from Top Personal Trainers

I0455132

Prince Point Publishing

DEDICATION

This book is dedicated to all of the incredible professionals and companies who took the time to submit content to this book. It has been a pleasure working with each of you, on the production of this book. The time you have all taken and the high quality content that you have all shared has truly gone above and beyond anything we could have ever expected when we first set out to publish this book. Thank you to everyone who made this possible.

PRINCE POINT PUBLISHING

Disclaimer

This book is an educational product that provides general health information. The materials in Unleash the Body Within are provided "as is" and without warranties of any kind either express or implied.

CONTENTS

ACKNOWLEDGMENTS

Austin Toloza – Condition & Competition Kickboxing
Sharon Adams - Rising Sun Fitness
Chris Pedroza – Supreme Assailant
Drew Dinwiddie – Drew Dinwiddie Personal Training
Jaymeson Anderson – Form & Function PT
Robert & Vicki Leasure – Spartan Training
Sergei Bakalov - Columbus Dance Centre
Andrew Johnston - Triumph Training
Michael Blauner – Personal Fitness by Michael Blauner

INTRODUCTION

If you've ever spent any amount of time strolling through the "Fitness & Nutrition" books section at your local book store, you've probably noticed one thing: there sure are a lot of books on the subject of losing weight and eating healthy. While this large amount of information on the subject may seem like a good thing, it could also be the one thing that keeps you from taking action towards your personal fitness and nutrition goals.

As you're probably aware, the fitness and nutrition industry is a multi-billion dollar industry. There are thousands upon thousands of people who rely on you to buy the next fitness book, exercise gadget, or DVD that hits the store shelves or the late night TV airwaves. Unfortunately, in this profit-driven world known as the fitness and nutrition industry, one priority gets lost: Getting real results for the end-user. You see, if one of these multi-million dollar companies actually produced a gadget or DVD that enabled everyone to be in the best shape of their lives forever, you wouldn't need to buy their products anymore - and that's exactly what they don't want to happen!

So what does this mean for you? Should you just throw in the towel and give up on any and all information out there? Of course not. You do, however, need to be more selective in where you get your information from.

The goal of this book was to interview real personal trainers who really train clients each and every day of their professional lives. Inside this book, you're not going to find interviews with celebrity fitness trainers. As you probably realize, most celebrity fitness trainers do very little day-to-day fitness training, because it conflicts with their schedules of book signings, producing DVDs, and filming television commercials. It's sad to say, but many great personal trainers stop being great personal trainers the moment they get "discovered" by the "machine" that is the fitness and nutrition's marketing industry.

Consider this book to be the opposite of those glitzy, celebrity-endorsed books. When we produced this book, we set out to find real world experts and that's exactly what we got. Our biggest challenge was getting these personal trainers to break away from their busy schedules of training their clients, so that they could actually share their advice in this book. The trainers who have contributed to this book "walk the walk", and the content they've provided, in the following chapters, reflects their true knowledge and expertise. So, without further ado, we present to you, the real world expert interviews!

1 AUSTIN TOLOZA

Condition and Competition Kickboxing
San Jose, CA
Head Strength and Conditioning Coach

My name is Austin Toloza and I am the Head Strength Coach at Condition and Competition Kickboxing located in San Jose, CA. We get people into shape through coaching kickboxing as well as strength and conditioning. Coach Ed Carpio is our Head Coach and has founded CCK after training and working with San Shou National Champion Cung Le.

Contact Information
Readers can contact me through my site http://www.Tolozastrength.com or by email at TolozaTraining@Gmail.com! You can also watch me at http://www.youtube.com/TolozaTrainer.

Is it true that exercise and a healthy diet can help reduce the chance of developing diabetes? If this is true, how can exercise and/or a good nutrition plan help prevent diabetes?

I believe an active life style along with a healthy diet can definitely reduce one's chances of developing diabetes. It's not some magical plan we came up with all of a sudden in order to combat this disease, it's really common sense. When one does physical activity, whether it is exercise or manual labor, they are utilizing calories and sugars that they have consumed. The problem is when people intake too much sugar, which is very common now, extra sugar that is left over may cause a variety of health problems.

Pairing physical activity with a healthy diet, or more specifically, a diet low on sugar, will only contribute to a healthy lifestyle and lessen one's chances in developing unnecessary complications with their diet.

Do people have to join the gym that their personal trainer belongs to, in order to hire them?

In some cases they do. Usually in these situations the personal trainer is legally obligated to only train clients under the "House Gym" which is the gym they work at. This is commonly seen in commercial health clubs such as 24, Club One, Bally's etc. Private studios who have trainers usually don't charge you membership.

What's a good way to find a reputable, trustworthy personal trainer?

Personal Trainers come a dime a dozen. The hard part is finding the trainers who really know their stuff as well as being passionate about their work! Word of mouth has always been a good way to learn about a trainer. If they created such an impression on someone that that person felt like they needed to tell you about their experience with him or her, that's genuine!

Also, look up their name online! If trainers are serious about what they do, they'll have some sort of web presence related to their profession. I have a Facebook page as well as a YouTube channel! This is because the Internet is such a growing resource that it should be taken advantage as a professional! Check if they have a blog, find out what their philosophy is, check service rating sites if they have profiles. You deserve every right to find out who is the best fit for you because this person will be affecting your life in one way, shape or form.

Are certain types of cardio workouts better than others?

Interval training really helps because you burn a lot of calories in a short amount of time. That type of work out gives you more bang for your buck! Other than that, any type of cardio work out is great as long as you enjoy doing it. It is very common for people to associate running with cardio; however any type of activity that gets your heart rate up and gets you moving for a prolonged period of time will do the trick! Things like playing basketball, soccer, tennis, swimming, doing a kickboxing class, Zumba class, conditioning class, intense yoga class or even that BUNS OF STEEL 1980's VHS tape you found in the storage bin will definitely help, as long as you enjoy what you are doing and do it consistently!

What's the difference between "aerobic" and "anaerobic" exercises?

I don't want to get all scientific on you so I will keep it simple. Aerobic exercise usually means you are doing an activity at a constant intensity for a time longer than 3 minutes. During these types of activities the body uses primarily oxygen. Anaerobic exercises are higher in intensity and shorter in duration. During these types of activities the body relies on other chemical reactions within the body instead of oxygen.

When thinking about aerobic exercises think about a marathon runner. When thinking about anaerobic exercises think about a sprinter.

Most experts seem to all agree that nuts are very healthy, but they seem to have a lot of fat in them. Won't eating high fat foods like nuts make it more difficult to lose weight?

This fear of fat is a horrible relic of the past that should die off just like the thigh master hype. Eating essential fats is good for your body because the human body can't create certain fats that it needs, so it must be consumed through the diet. The problem occurs when people eat too many carbs, which if not utilized, will turn into fat.

You burn fat when you sleep; that is a fact not an opinion, so that whole fat burning zone is bogus. Any fat free products are also bogus, because if you take out fat from a food it becomes tasteless since our bodies are built to love the taste of fat, which makes companies put more sugars in these products to compensate for the taste.

Bottom line; don't be afraid of fats, just moderate your carbohydrate, sugar intake and watch your calories.

How long should people rest in between workouts?

People who are just starting to work out should leave a day between work out days to get their bodies and nervous system acclimated. Many people go all out 5 days a week only to burn out after week 2. Don't be that person. If your goal is weight loss, hard work out days can be followed by a day of light activity and reduced calorie intake.

You are a fool to think you can go 5 days a week hard and keep it up for more than 3 months. Your body needs time to grow lean body mass and reduce fat mass as needed to compensate for the increased activity and reduced calories. Your nervous system also needs to rest if it's constantly under stress. If one doesn't rest, they don't give their body a chance to do its job! Like I always say to my clients, rest is where the magic happens following a work out.

Should children lift weights?

There have been studies that say that children who weight lift can do it safely without it really affecting them in a negative way, however personally I believe that children shouldn't for one simple reason; they will get bored out of their minds! When you were a kid, was your idea of fun lifting a dumbbell? Most likely not!

You can create the most safest and effective weight lifting program ever, but it won't mean anything if the person doesn't want to do it. In my experience, all kids want to do is play. Play, play, play! Their minds formulate unlimited possibilities on what they should be doing, and I guarantee you lifting weights are not one of them.

The best way to get a kid in shape is to play with them!

Who should the average person talk to about which exercise program would be best for them?

Their personal doctor is one person that can definitely point them in the right direction. Their doctor usually has a medical history and knows what to advise that person to do, and with that knowledge, that person can take it to a Personal Trainer or an Exercise Physiologist and get their advice on which exercise program best suits their personal needs.

Going to the buffest guy at the gym for advice may seem easier, and I'm sure they have some awesome advice, however they lack the critical medical information and health history your doctor knows, which means what worked for them, may not work for you.

Should a personal trainer know all of the medications someone is on? Why or why not?

YES! As a personal trainer, we're not going to know what every medication does, however it is our responsibility to find out their side effects related to physical activity if our clients are on any of them.

If someone is taking beta-blockers for example, the trainer has to be aware that their client's heart rate may be lower than usual, as well as their blood pressure. People who are on statins to lower their cholesterol may have muscle aches or become nauseated at time. It is essential that a Personal Trainer know these things about their client so they can know how to adjust their work out session and program accordingly.

How important is nutrition if someone works out consistently?

Nutrition is 70% and exercise is 30% of overall body change. No matter how much you exercise, if you are not ingesting proper nutrition, your body change and performance will be minimal at best.

I'll use the good 'ole race horse example. If you had a race horse, and your living was based on how much that race horse won, would you feed it cheap crap, or the highest quality food you can get your hands on?

Chances are you would probably be more mindful of what that horse ate and even feed it food that is specifically nutritious for that horse. People should treat themselves the same, because their lives also depend on it.

Is it a good idea to workout when feeling mentally stressed? Why or why not?

Yes! If you are feeling mentally stressed, doing a workout will help you unleash all that tension as well as release endorphins within your body. These hormones make you feel so good. You may be stressed, but when it comes to working out, it's your time, and if you push yourself in that work out, you may feel better leaving the gym than coming into it!

Is it safe for obese people to lift weights?

When I have obese clients, I always start them off moving their own body weight, period. I will add some light weights here and there, but I would never have an obese person back squatting 135 pounds. If they're over 350 pounds and not an NFL lineman, it doesn't make sense to me to make them lift and additional 135lbs when they can barely sit down and stand up.

Body weight exercises are a must for obese people. They are safe and more efficient.

Should women lift weights if they don't want to get bulky looking? If yes, how can they lift weights and not get that bulky/masculine look?

This whole "I just want tone" thing is a result of not knowing the facts and relying on advertisement and media to drive one's perspective on what something "should" be rather than what something really is.

Women lack the hormones to get really "bulky/masculine" looking. Men get bulkier easily because their testosterone levels are higher as opposed to their women counterparts. Women who feel like they bulk easier when they lift weights may need to check their diets.

Women who do compound lifts with moderate weight should be fine, as long as you are doing it safely and efficiently.

Is it true that some people naturally lose weight faster than others? Why or why not is this the case?

Everyone is built differently. A person who has Eskimo ancestry is built differently than a person who has African ancestry. Their ancestors grew up in different environments, which mean their bodies and diets developed differently. It can be easier for one person to lose weight faster than another because that is how their bodies were built, however that shouldn't discourage those who lose weight a slower pace.

As long as you get to your end result, you will be the winner. It's not about who gets there first, it's just about who finally gets there!

2 SHARON ADAMS

Rising Sun Fitness
Reston, VA
Owner

Rising Sun Fitness, LLC is my personal fitness training company. I do one on one training with people at all levels of fitness, triathlon and run coaching, bootcamp classes, yoga, kid's yoga and fitness classes, etc.

Contact Information
Sharon@risingsunfitness.com
703.796.9282

What are some questions that people should ask a personal trainer before hiring them?

The more information a client can give to their prospective trainer before working out with them is quite helpful. In this regard, the trainer will sometimes almost be able to already have a feel for how the first workout together should be structured and can plan the best. The client should ask the trainer about their expectations of the client, if they have experience working with any injuries that they have, and it is great if they can talk to a past client to hear firsthand any recommendations. It is also helpful to ask the trainer if they give the client workouts to do on their own before the next session together- some trainers do and some do not.

Are there ways to reduce recovery time or soreness between workouts, without taking supplements?

Absolutely- the more you move while sore, the better recovery your sore muscles will have. The repetitive, low impact moving of the muscles allows increased blood flow to those working muscles, bringing to it oxygen and other nutrients for recovery. In addition, hydrating, having Vitamin C as well as a carbohydrate protein snack of at least 200 calories immediately after a highly intense workout sets you up for the best recovery. Light stretching or yoga, legs up the wall position, and adequate sleep and rest are also helpful for recovery.

What are some ways to verify the credentials/certifications of a personal trainer?

To some level you will have to trust that the trainer has the certifications that they say they have. I am biased, but I recommend someone who has a college DEGREE in the fitness/exercise physiology background.

Why don't crash diets work?

Any diet that someone cannot follow for every single day of their lifetime will not work. I tell my clients to never eat in one day in a way they could not sustain forever.

If someone feels that their trainer is pushing them too hard, or not hard enough how should they handle this?

They should speak openly to the trainer and let them know their feelings, as well as listen to the communication from the trainer. There is a give and take here. Goals may need to be amended if the client isn't comfortable or doesn't have the desire to work intensely at some points.

How does someone tone up and lose fat under their arms and around their triceps?

To lose fat, you would need to take in less calories than you expend. You cannot spot reduce, so you cannot selectively lose the fat in the triceps area, however you can TONE this area. To tone the triceps, you can do any exercise or movement including elbow extension such as pushups and dips off of a stair or chair. That being said, for the biggest complaint of women..... it is readily available to work on it—you don't need any equipment to do pushups or dips! Other exercises are triceps pushdowns with a cable, dumbbell triceps kickbacks, overhead French press, "skullcrushers" and many more.

For people who are always tired, won't working out make them feel like they have even less energy?

I guarantee anyone who begins working out with me, if this is their worry, a money back guarantee that they will feel more energized if they follow a correct exercise AND nutrition program!
What's the difference between "good carbs" and "bad carbs"?

Good carbs are whole grains, fruit, vegetables, beans and low fat dairy. These are all nutrient rich sources of calories that have good amounts of carbohydrates/energy within them. "Bad" carbs are nutrient poor food refined grains. These include sweets, white breads, cakes, cookies, sodas, etc. These are digested quickly and cause a spike in blood sugars.

Fish seems to have a lot of fat in it. Will people gain weight if they eat too much fish?

This would depend on so many factors, such as: how is the fish cooked, what is the portion/amount that they are eating. Fish has good fat, however, if it is cooked in an unhealthy way, and eaten with other high fat things, then this would not be healthy and you could gain or not lose weight. It is recommended to eat fish 2x/week and not more because of the high mercury content in some fish.

If someone is a heavy smoker, should their workout routine be adjusted at all? If so, how?

If someone is a heavy smoker, even more important than exercise is that they stop smoking immediately.

What are the biggest mistakes people make when hiring a personal trainer?

The biggest mistake people make in hiring a personal trainer is in thinking that the work is done! Sometimes they think that just by meeting with a trainer, they will become lean! They need to work hard while there... then they need to go home and live a healthy lifestyle and follow direction of their trainer, and be back again when they say they will!

What can people do to avoid back injuries when they're lifting weights?

You shouldn't injure your back when lifting weights if you are lifting with proper form, an appropriate amount for your fitness level, and holding correct posture when lifting. Correct posture means a neutral spine (not excessively arched or rounded) with the abdominal muscles engaged. This does not mean sucking the stomach in, as some people will think. Engaging the abdominal muscles is a similar feeling to "bracing" or turning the muscles "on" as if someone were trying to push you over and you were trying to not allow them to move you.

3 CHRIS PEDROZA

Supreme Assailant

El Paso, TX

CEO/Instructor

If you are an athlete OR unhappy average Joe looking for faster results than the "NORM" in the greater EL PASO area, who wants to improve your performance, an adult who wants to lose weight, gain muscle, increase your cardiorespiratory endurance and muscular endurance, have FUN when you exercise, or a combat athlete who wants to step in the cage to achieve an overall greater VO2 Max, I will guarantee your results OR DOUBLE YOUR MONEY BACK!

As the owner of SUPREME ASSAILANT, my philosophy blends ideas from the disciplines of exercise science, coaching and athletic skill development to design and implement protocols for athletes, adults as well as children of any age.

MY belief is simple: Show up and I'll do the rest! Results are in direct proportion to your commitment, attendance, discipline and correct nutritional intake in following the guidance and direction of the program.

MY diverse list of clientele include youth through collegiate athletes mixing with firefighters, Conditioning Camp participants, business professionals, Jiu-Jitsu and Full Contact Fighters and competitive bodybuilders, to name a few.

MY training invites you to step "outside the comfort zone" of traditional programming and find out what it really means to TRAIN! "TWICE THE RESULTS, HALF THE TIME OR DOUBLE YOUR MONEY BACK"

I welcome the opportunity to earn your business. On behalf of myself, thank you for your interest.

COMMITTED TO YOUR SUCCESS,

CHRIS PEDROZA
OWNER/INSTRUCTOR OF SUPREME ASSAILANT
www.supremeassailant.net
supremeassailant@gmail.com
(Athletic Conditioning Specialist, Body-weight Training Specialist, Nutrition Specialist, Muay Thai Instructor, Health & Fitness Article Contributor for MMARECRUITER.COM (Mike Zuccerello), and Health & Fitness Correspondent for FUERTEMEN.COM (Sidney Alvarez)

What are the best foods that people should eat to gain energy and why are these foods so important?

Blueberries, Beans, Cantaloupe, Strawberries, Mango, Spinach, Salmon, Nuts, Tea, Tomatoes, Soy, Low fat dairy products, Oatmeal, Whole grains, Citrus fruit, Peppers, Sweet potatoes. The carbohydrates, proteins, and fats in food provide calories to fuel exercise and energize your body. Contrary to myth, vitamins and minerals do not themselves provide any energy. (They are, however, involved in the process of converting nutrients into fuel for energy and are an important part of a healthy diet.)

Is it better to lift weights with free weights or with weight machines? Why is one better than the other?

General Fitness: Machines can give you a great foundation for general strength training, whether you're just starting out or aren't sure what your goals should be.

Functional Fitness: If you exercise to improve your ability to move and function in everyday life, then free weights will be a better choice because you can use them to mimic normal movement patterns, making them easier over time.

Muscle size and strength: Machines usually win in this case because they can really target and isolate a single muscle group while allowing you to lift more weight, which is crucial for developing size and strength. But ideally, a combination of free weights and machines will help build strength and size.

Is it true that eating too many vegetables will make most people gain water weight?

It's virtually impossible to gain weight eating vegetables only, unless you are cooking them in a lot of fat, or adding other ingredients to them. The amount you would need to eat to create a calorie surplus would result in feeling impossibly stuffed.

How can someone do resistance training if they don't own weights or belong to a gym?

Do some push-ups: Depending on your fitness level, you can do them standing and facing a wall, on the floor with your knees bent, or on the floor with your legs straight and toes touching the ground.

Try seated rows: Sitting on the floor with your legs straight, wrap an old T-shirt or stretchy exercise band behind the soles of your feet. With one end in each hand, squeeze your shoulder blades together by bringing your elbows behind you while stretching the T-shirt or band. Return to the starting position.

Work your arms with dips: With the palms of your hands on a chair or bench and your feet on the floor, scoot your rear end off the end of the chair. Bend your elbows, lowering your body, then straighten your arms to return to the starting position. Pick up some dumbbells or use makeshift weights, such as water-filled milk jugs, soup cans, water bottles, or filled plastic or cloth grocery bags (with handles).

Shrug with shoulder raises: With or without weights in your hands, raise your shoulders up toward your ears, hold, then relax.

Opt for the shoulder press: With a weight in each hand, bring your hands up to ear level with your arms forming 90-degree angles at the elbow for the starting position. Straighten your arms above your head. Return your hands to their starting position.

Do some lateral raises: Holding weights by your side, raise both arms out to the side no higher than shoulder height. Slowly lower.

Be creative with bicep curls: Holding a filled grocery bag in each hand, arms and elbows tucked in by your sides, bend your elbows, bringing your hands up toward your shoulders with your palms facing you. Slowly return your hands down by your sides.

Get down with crunches: Lying on your back with your knees bent, reach for your knees, hold for two counts, then return to the floor.

Do people really lose muscle as they get older? If so, how much muscle do they lose on average, and can anything be done to slow down this process?

Muscles take longer to respond to brain signals in your 50's than they did in your 20's. As a normal course of aging, you begin to lose the muscle fibers that are responsible for making you move quickly. The speed of transmission of impulses from the brain to the muscles also slows down, so it takes longer to get the signal. Your muscles also can't repair themselves as quickly as they used to, due to a decrease in enzyme activities and protein turnover.

How can someone figure out how many calories they should be eating each day?

The number of calories that you should eat depends of your weight, age, height, your activity levels and whether you are trying to lose, maintain or gain weight. You need balance the calories that you take each day in the diet with the calories that you expend each day.

Is it true that muscle will turn to fat if someone stops working out?

Muscle will never turn into fat simply because they are not the same cells. If your eating habits remain the same as it was when you were training, you will put on more weight thus giving the look that your muscles turned to fat, because your not burning the same amount of calories like you were when you were working out.

What is "body fat percentage"? How does this differ from "body mass index"?

BMI is the body mass index. If you are an athlete or active, you are going to have more weight in muscle than the average person, and your BMI may not accurately reflect your health and fitness, or how healthy and fit you look.

This is where body fat percentage comes in. Body fat percentage is literally measuring what percentage of your body is made up of fat. Everything else is usually referred to as "lean tissue." This gives a more accurate representation of health, fitness and leanness for someone who is physically active.

What can thin people do to build muscle?

The first thing you need to do when setting up a regime for weight and muscle gain is that as a skinny guy with a fast metabolism you need to eat more! Not just a little bit more but you need to consume more of the things you really need to gain muscle which is calories and protein.

The problem most skinny people have with this is that they become too full too quickly before they can ingest the required calories, which is why you need to pick and choose your foods carefully. It is recommended that you eat calorie dense food that does not fill you up as much but are bursting with energy such as: Avocado, Whole Eggs, Tuna & Salmon in Olive Oil, Rice, Pasta, Potatoes.

Can couples or groups of people workout with a personal trainer at the same time?

Yes, simple. The couple that plays together stays together. Exercising with your partner will strengthen your muscles, your heart, and your relationship.

If someone hasn't worked out in years, how should they get started in the safest way possible?

Any form of regular exercise, together with a healthy and nutritious diet should help you to lose weight. Start walking - outside is better than a treadmill if possible. Start off with maybe 10 minutes and increase your time/distance every day or so until you are walking further and faster. Diet - well, lots of fruit, vegetables etc. and cut out all fizzy sugary drinks and sweets and biscuits etc. Just start gently and keep at it. You should tone up quite quickly and then start losing weight. But it won't happen overnight.

Is it safe to workout first thing in the morning, on an empty stomach?

Do NOT exercise on an empty stomach. The theory that you burn more fat with no available blood sugar is a myth. In fact, it can result in the loss of muscle tissue. So, make sure to get a healthy snack in you about 45 minutes before you train.

Do personal trainers usually have insurance?
Every time you train, instruct, or consult with any of your clients, there is risk involved. As a professional in your field, you need to practice loss prevention daily by serving the needs of your clients in a safe environment. You need to protect yourself by purchasing quality insurance.

How can people, with very busy work schedules and family commitments, fit working out into their schedule?

When you work out you will feel good about yourself and your body. This, in turn, will make you more productive and efficient in your work and with your family. So, if you're busy, remember, "Who isn't?" Don't let it be your excuse. There is always something you can do, even if it's a little bit at a time. This is the simple choice each of us must make on a daily basis and don't forget: even five minutes can get you very, very far.

How many grams of fat should people consume each day, if they want to lose weight?

The amount of fat you really need per day is quite low only about 10 or 20 grams. To keep the fat in your diet to a reasonable level, consider reducing the high fat foods you eat (high fat meats, desserts, fried foods, and spreads). A reasonable serving of meat is 3-4 ounces, about the size of a deck of cards. And we really can get enough fat in our diet without frying foods or adding mounds of butter and other sauces. Aim for less than 30% of your calories from fat and you'll be getting just the right balance for your best health.

PRINCE POINT PUBLISHING

4 DREW DINWIDDIE

Drew Dinwiddie Personal Training

Atlanta, GA

Owner/Trainer

Drew Dinwiddie Personal Training (DDPT.COM) has been operating out of midtown Atlanta since 2003. Active in nutrition as well as strength and endurance training for more than 10 years, Drew Dinwiddie has received local and national media attention for his ability to create effective and unique fitness and nutrition programs based on the needs of any individual. Working with a diverse range of clients – from athletes working to build muscle mass and endurance, to busy professionals seeking a healthier lifestyle and a leaner look – he is known for his professionalism, ability to motivate and his genuine passion for helping clients reach their fitness goals.

Dinwiddie earned a bachelor of arts degree in communications from the College of Charleston and is certified by the National Strength and Conditioning Association (NSCA-CPT) , the American Council on Exercise (ACE) and the National Council on Certified Personal Training (NCCPT) and by the American Red Cross in CPR. He participates in continuing education courses year-round.

How does someone know how hard to push themselves when they're working out?

A heart rate monitor is a great way to keep track of your exertion during a session. A trainer can help you determine a healthy zone to stay in for the session.

If someone just recently had surgery can they lift weights or workout? What should be taken into consideration in these situations?

This depends on the nature of the surgery. A qualified personal trainer will ask the client to follow their physician's orders and to receive written clearance to begin or continue to fitness routine following a medical procedure.

Is it possible to lose fat and gain muscle at the same time? If so, how can this be done effectively?

Yes. A regimen of resistance training and endurance training can produce these results. Nutrition must be closely monitored to unsure that calories are weighted properly between fat, carbohydrates, and protein.

If someone has been a "yo-yo dieter" their entire lives, how can a personal trainer help people like this?

A qualified personal trainer will identify the flaws in someone's approach to dieting and offer suggestions/guidelines for improvement. Often people adhere to "fad" diets when what they really need is to be empowered with some very basic knowledge of nutrition and how to properly fuel their bodies. I try to teach people how to make healthy nutrition a part of their life rather than a "diet" which has a starting and ending point.

What is the difference between a "high impact" and a "low impact" workout?

Examples of High impact exercises are running, jumping, punching, jumping rope and plyometrics. Low impact exercises include walking, biking, hiking and swimming to name a few. High impact movements should only be performed by people who already have a basic fitness level established. There is greater risk of injury to the knees, ankles, hips and back. Low impact movements are a great place to start for beginners or for older individuals who are at risk for already having joint disease or osteoporosis.

How much of a say should the client have in determining which exercises they do?

The client and trainer need to have open communication and a good trainer is able to determine how hard to push a client. Some clients just don't "like" certain exercises but at the end of the session or after achieving a weight loss goal will admit that it was necessary and that they were glad we performed them. If there is a legitimate medical excuse or reason to discontinue or avoid certain exercises they must be avoided.

Why do certain "non-fat" foods still make people gain weight?

Fat is gained based on a "calories in vs. calories out" model. If a client is consuming more calories than are being expended they will gain weight. If they create a deficit in calories they will lose weight. A calorie deficit is created by consuming fewer calories and performing exercise to burn more.

Is it true that some exercises produce results faster than others? If so, which exercises provide the best and worst "returns on investment"?

Sure - does high intensity cardio activity produce faster results than wrist curls? The most appropriate exercises are dependent on the fitness level and the goals of the client. If a client's goal is weight loss the suggestion by his/her trainer would be different from those given to a client who is interested in gaining muscle mass.

How should someone determine how many grams of protein and carbs they should be eating each day?

This again is determined by the goal of the client and can only be determined by working with your trainer on an individual basis. The total number of calories suggested for intake differs from person to person and so, too, does the suggested number calories from carbs/fat and protein.

Is it a good idea for someone to work out if they have a cold?

Depending on the severity of the cold it's likely not a problem to workout with one. It is however inconsiderate to go to the gym if you think you are contagious. I instruct my clients to see if they feel like working out - and then decide if it's best that they come in for a lower intensity workout that day. Often it would be a workout that I write for them via email so they can go at their own pace and can call it quits if they begin to feel sick without having to use one of their paid sessions with me.

Is it better to exercise every part of the body on the same day, or it better to focus on different muscle groups on different days? Please explain why one is better than the other.

The answer depends on a client's goals. An obese person who needs to loose 50lbs should likely start by simply walking on the treadmill 2-3 times a week. Someone in moderate physical condition seeking to tone up and lose a little fat might start a program of cardio three times a week and resistance training two times a week and the bodybuilder who wants to gain muscle mass might spend an entire workout of arms, or legs, or back , or core.

Another consideration is how much time can be allotted to the gym or to working out. If a five day a week program can be implemented it gives the trainer many more options in terms of how to split the workouts

If someone doesn't have the time to spend hours cooking healthy meals, how can they still eat healthy?

Yes, it is more challenging to eat healthy without cooking at home but it can be done. It's important to make healthy choices when eating at a restaurant and learn what foods/dishes to stay away from.

What should a personal trainer take into consideration when working with each individual client?

A trainer must always keep the clients goals in mind. It is important to meet with the client, make sure you both understand that you are working toward the same goal and to propose a plan to the client to achieve that goal.

If someone isn't sore after a workout, does that mean they didn't work out hard enough?

No - it means that they may not have performed any new movements that session. Muscle soreness is created by tiny tears in the muscle and must be given adequate time to heal. Some soreness is expected but is certainly not the measure of a "good workout".

For more information visit DDPT.COM

5 JAYMESON ANDERSON

Form & Function Personal Training

Chicago, IL

Owner

Form&Function Personal Training, Chicago was established in 2007 as a client service determined to better educate and communicate with individuals being trained. F&F also serves to reach out to people with the desire and potential to make a serious lifestyle change. You are invited to come see for yourself at www.formandfunctiontraining.com

Get Form. Get Function. Get in the best shape of your life.

What should people look out for when hiring a personal trainer?

There are the obvious elements such as education, experience, and technical ability, but don't forget that you will be spending a lot of time with this person, and it is important to feel a sense of trust and "personal" involvement when you are in the company of your trainer/trainer to be. He/she should truly care about producing a result for you, and will be accompanying you through a legitimately difficult process, so take care to choose a trainer who is a true leader.

If someone has a friend who is in good shape, who is willing to give them exercise advice, why is it still a good idea to hire a personal trainer?

A truly effective personal training service must provide a multi-faceted approach that includes much more than just technical advice about resistance and endurance training. Motivation, coaching, testing, accountability (getting you to the gym every time), dietary guidance and consultation, "homework" routine design, physical therapy, as well as the development of flexibility, posture, and balance are a few of the necessary benefits that your friend may or may not be able to provide. As I've always told people: "There are several areas of focus when creating a comprehensive change in the body. A weak link in the process can potentially lead to failure."

Is it true that people should take periods of time off from working out? If so, how long should these "workout vacations" last and how frequently should they occur?

The amount or recovery time needed it contingent upon the frequency, volume, weight, speed, and rest periods specific to the exercise prescription of that individual. It is very important to recover tissue that has been stressed and broken down during exercise, however, the above factors, as well as age, gender, lifestyle, and exercise type must be taken into account before making a decision.

What are some tips to help people stick with an exercise program and not quit?

You must consider this a "long term" investment of time, effort, and discomfort in an effort to achieve optimum health and a better looking and functioning body. If it took a significant amount of time to "de-train" and/or gain body fat, it will take a comparable amount of time to reduce the fat, and bring your conditioning levels back up. Those who expect an immediate result will be disappointed. Those who consider this a lifestyle change, and ready to make a life-long commitment will have greater success.

What is a "drop set"?

A drop-set is a set in which you start the movement at a heavier weight, and "drop" the weight (a percentage specific to your routine prescription) when you begin to fatigue. You immediately continue on at a lower weight until fatigued again. You can drop weight once or several times within a drop-set.

If someone likes to listen to music, on a personal music player with headphones, when

they workout, is this considered rude by most personal trainers?

Not rude, but rather, ridiculous. If you're hiring someone just to carry your weights, and sit there silently watching you work out, you need a porter not a trainer.

Which types of people can benefit the most from a personal trainer?

Those that truly want change for themselves. Those individuals that come in the door ready to work, and truly want to gain or re-gain control over their bodies will find that they are able to increase muscle and ability as well as lose fat faster. We can spend time motivating you (and we're pretty good at it), but that is time that could be spent exercising...if you're coming in the door prepared mentally, you will accomplish more physically.

What are "boot camps" and why are they so popular?

Fitness boot camps are quite similar to the military boot camps that they take their name from. They are "camps" that offer fully controlled environments designed to remove ones control, or lack thereof. They teach you how to eat and exercise, while keeping you away from poor foods, and holding you accountable for your workouts. They are becoming popular because a large number of people in the United States have had a lack of success on their own, or even with a personal trainer. The problem being that they cannot control themselves, and their trainer cannot go home with them from the gym and help affect their decisions. The camp solves that problem.

How can people overcome junk food cravings?

I've always thought it was harder to try to eat junk food sparingly, and easier not to buy it in the first place. This works well at home, but when you're at the office or out with friends, try comparing the amount of calories within the food you're craving to the amount of time you would need to spend exercising to burn off those calories. When you consider that 2 minutes of pleasure from a sweet/fatty snack could require 45 minutes of jogging on the treadmill, the snack no longer seems so appealing.

Do most personal trainers yell at people, like drill sergeants, to keep them motivated? What if someone wants to hire a personal trainer without being screamed at?

Actually, this in not very common at all. I consider myself an exceptionally tough trainer, and I rarely use a loud tone of voice with my clients. Those that need to be "yelled" at, usually aren't ready for this process, and need either a boot camp setting, or some additional time to prepare mentally before returning to the training sessions. This process is like a college classroom...the professor wants to keep people calm and quiet so that he/she can teach them more with less wasted time and distraction. Fitness and diet instruction is similar. A certain amount of coaching and motivation is essential, but it you're kicking and screaming, and want to leave, you should do just that, and return when you are ready to focus and learn.

How does someone know if they're "over-training"?

Signs of overtraining are chronic fatigue, interrupted sleep patterns, diminished returns (loss of strength/speed), chronic soreness, and stress injuries. Breaking down the muscle is only half the battle...rest and nutrition are required to repair and strengthen the body so that it is adequately prepared for the next workout. Proceeding with exercise before full recovery can lead to overtraining, and it's more common than you'd think.

How will a trainer know what program is right for their client?

Proper assessment, testing, and consultation. You should never accept the services of a trainer that writes you generic and/or repetitive exercise routines. Each routine should be tailored to the specific needs of the individual, period.

Is it typically acceptable for people to bring their children to a personal training session?

This depends on the gym. My current gym has the space and services to accommodate children safely. Some of the gyms I've worked at in the past were not prepared for kids, and I felt that it was a danger to the parent/client as well as the child for them to be present.

How much sleep should people get when they exercise regularly?

I've always recommended 8-10 un-interrupted hours if possible.

Is it customary for a personal trainer to provide references of satisfied clients?

Providing a reference for the client to contact is not a common pre-requisite, but I think it could be a good idea. I do however have several testimonials on my own website, and most trainers will list these within their print material and on their websites as a way for prospective clients to see the comments of past clients. Beware though; I would imagine that most of my trainers wouldn't list a bad testimonial...

jaymeson@formandfunctiontraining.com
847-757-2284

6 ROBERT & VICKI LEASURE

Spartan Training

Chandler AZ

Owners

Robert is ISSA Certified and Vicki is S.M.A.R.T Certified. Both Vicki and Robert share a passion for personal training and have a lifetime of experience in weight loss, exercise, fitness and nutrition. Robert and Vicki having logged in well over 20,000 hours of Personal Training experience, and are both qualified Master Trainers and Fitness Experts.

Robert currently writes health and fitness articles and has written fitness articles for a local Prime Times News Magazine. Robert also is an Expert, with published health and fitness articles at Self Growth.

Robert has published blog sites on, Nutrition...Health...Resistance Training...Weight Loss...and a bi monthly Spartan Newsletter...

Robert has mastered a 12 year study in Siddha Yoga, along with a study in the teachings of J. Krishnamurti. Many of these studies involve a realized understanding in relation to the philosophy of the mind. Over the years Robert has developed a working understanding of how to effectively apply these teachings to the psychology of weight loss and fitness, and in relation to helping clients reach their weight loss and fitness goals. Robert applies vision and affirmation techniques that enable the re-programing of the sub-conscious mind, in which fear doubt and anxiety about weight loss are replaced with a positive integration of health and fitness into the client's lifestyle.

Vicki is an accomplished female bodybuilder and enjoys staying fit and exercising. With Robert as her coach, Vicki at the age of 52, Vicki competed in her first NPC Female Bodybuilding contest. She won first place in the Master's division, the Heavyweight division, and the Overall, giving her the title of Ms. NPC Western Regional 2007.

At the age of 53 she went on to win the 2008 Arizona NPC Master's, Heavyweight, and Over-all, giving her the title of Ms. NPC Arizona 2008. Vicki followed those wins up with placing 5th in the Heavyweight division of the NPC USA Female Bodybuilding Competition in 2009.

Robert also developed "The Spartan Training System" (STS) As a Qualified Fitness Expert and Certified Personal Trainer with well over 20,000 hours of Personal Training experience; The Spartan Training System is one of the most effective and efficient Personal Training Systems, I have ever developed, to help clients reach their Weight loss and Fitness goals. With the Spartan Training System, you will immediately begin to lose body fat and unwanted pounds, gain Muscle tone, and improve overall Health and appearance. As a Spartan Client you will be completely revitalized with this unique approach, of transforming both body and mind. With the Spartan

Training System you will achieve real, long lasting results, and create a permanent condition where weight gain is no longer an issue. To integrate Health and Fitness into your Lifestyle, you must do more than exercise your body. You must Exercise the Mind as well. The Spartan Training System will teach you how to integrate Health and Fitness into your Lifestyle, through changing your perceptions and attitude toward Exercise, Fitness, Nutrition and Health. I will not only show you the correct Physical Exercise and Conditioning Techniques. I will teach you the techniques that will help you re-program the sub-consciousness mind with positive thoughts. I will inspire you to Exercise determination and maintain Motivation. Breaking bad habits is one of the most challenging things that one can face. Together, we will replace bad habits with good ones. You will develop and integrate healthy habits that uplift your spirit and bring you happiness through fitness, healthy living, and energized mental clarity.

Does weight training cause people to lose flexibility?

No...Weight Training increases flexibility. When exercising you must move into the full stretch position to fully activate muscle fiber. Most people don't even know what the stretch positions are for each exercise. So it is that when exercising correctly you are actually increasing flexibility.

If someone can only work-out once a week, should they even bother?

Yes. Exercising once a week can help improve strength, endurance, flexibility, cardio-vascular health, improve well-being, and increase metabolism.

Other than losing weight and gaining muscle, what are some of the other benefits of getting in shape?

There are many benefits, which I named in question '2'.

What can people do if they "plateau" and stop seeing results from their workout routine?

Find a new trainer. No just kidding...there are many things you can do to transcend the limitations of the human condition. Just to name a few...foremost would be to increase intensity, increase the of volume of training (which include increasing weight or increasing reps and or sets), also nutrition and supplementation are important to consider as well as sleep.

Is it a bad idea to eat right after working out? Why or why not?

Well that depends on what you eat. The best time for protein synthesis for muscle repair is right after exercise. Studies reveal that after exercise, there is nothing more effective for protein synthesis for muscle repair than isolate whey protein. The reason why? Right after resistance training an anabolic window opens for about 30 minutes. Basically what this means is that muscle cells are open and fat cells are closed. This is optimal time for protein synthesis for muscle repair. An isolate whey protein drink is the best choice after your workout.

What should someone do if they get muscle cramps during a workout? Should they work through it or do something else?

When you get muscle cramps you should stop exercising and take steps to get rid of the muscle cramp. Set one...walk it off. If that doesn't work try stretching if away. If that doesn't work apply a heating pad to the cramping area. If that doesn't work the best cure on the planet for muscle cramps is pickle brine. Yes that's right, pickle juice. They even make sports drinks with pickle brine in it to stop cramping. Pickle juice stops cramps dead in their tracks; usually in about one minute the cramp will disappear.

How can someone tell if their personal trainer's certification is legitimate?

Personal Training Certifications all have a certification number on them along with an expiration date along with the name of the company...ISSA or NASM or ACE or etc. Just write down the certification number and call the certification company and inquire if the name on the certificate is legitimate and if the number is valid and or expired.

Is there any true benefit to warming up, cooling down, or stretching before or after exercising? If there is, why are these things important?

Yes. Warm up before exercise and stretch after. Warming up before exercise increases blood flow heart rate and flexibility. Warming up also increases neuromuscular connection, thereby reducing the risk of injury during exercise. Stretching after exercise increases flexibility, and also helps the body to remove metabolites out of the exercised muscles, which will help reduce DOMS (Delayed Onset Muscle Soreness).

Why is it important for people to work on improving their balance and how can they do this?

Balance is important to maintain throughout life. Without balance you are simply more inclined to injury. A balanced body is a balanced mind. A balanced body and mind are in direct relation to balanced health. The best way to improve balance - hatha yoga is a great place to start. Hatha yoga improves balance mind, body, spirit. A wholeness of balance is achieved through breathing properly while stretching, harmonizing the central nervous system, respiratory system, and the circulatory system. Improving mental clarity, the immune system, the glandular system, and the digestive system...all of which relates to optimal health.

What are some of the most common myths about losing weight?

The HCG Diet is the latest myth about losing weight. I always say you cannot starve fat off; you have to burn it off. The only thing you starve off is your lean muscle, lowering the metabolism resulting in gaining more fat weight. Fad diets are leading the way in myth building and Exercise infomercials are neck and neck with Exercise gadgets.

What is the correct way to breathe when working out?

An easy way to understand how to breathe correctly is to think of exertion as outward, breathe outward. When you are exerting your muscles, exhale. The inward breath is always at the end of the exertion, breathe inward, inhale.

If a particular exercise hurts, is that normal?

If exercise hurts then yes it is normal. If an exercise hurts as in injures then no it is not normal. Pain resulting from exercise is normal because blood occlusion is painful and lactic acid build up are painful. Think of it like this; if the pain is in the muscle then it is a good pain; if the pain is in the joint then it is a bad pain

Footnote: Is injury during exercise normal? Yes. When we exercise we tear our muscles. They are called micro tears which are actually muscle cells torn in two. When this happens insulin growth factor one is released to repair the micro tears. The IGF 1 aka stem cell are like a drops of oil... and drop onto the torn muscle cells and this creates new muscle cells and this is how we increase lean muscle. One cell gets torn in two and IGF 1 creates another two cell out of the split fiber.

985 W. Chandler Heights Rd Suite 12
Chandler AZ 85248
http://Spartan-Training.com

480-802-2222
ChandlerFitness@Spartan-Training.com

7 SERGEI BAKALOV

Sergei Bakalov

Columbus Dance Centre

Columbus, OH

Personal Trainer/Dance Instructor/Healthy Lifestyle Consultant

Since opening in October 2002, Columbus Dance Centre has been providing quality dance, fitness and music instruction to students of all ages. Columbus Dance Centre uses dance and music to train confident, articulate and intelligent young persons. By building the ability to learn, think and act in an athletically artistic environment our program yields both a talented dancer and a highly successful individual. Columbus Dance Centre's experienced faculty addresses the physical, intellectual and emotional elements of a student's being in an age-specific manner.

Why is it so important to drink water and how much water should people drink each day?

Over 60% of the human body contains water and any physical activities including everyday stuff like walking, talking running etc. make us lose water by sweating it out. In order not to dehydrate, feel and stay healthy we have to replace lost water by consuming about 8 glasses of water per day. More active you are the more water you have to drink. Plus don't forget that water flushes out bad toxins.

Does it make a difference if someone just does all of their exercise over the weekend as compared to spreading it out over the week?

It depends on what the personal goals of this person are. This is very individual. Different exercise programs can be tailored for different goals. Generally, if you're just looking to get your muscles in tone even exercising once a week can be very beneficial.

How often should someone workout with a personal trainer?

Working out with a personal trainer is always specific to the individual. Generally, for an average person without any knowledge in exercising I recommend having workouts with a personal trainer every time you are in the gym for first 3 months. Then maybe 1-2 times a week for next 6 months. Then maybe 1 a week for the rest of your workout program until you get the desired results.

Is coffee bad for someone who's trying to lose weight or get in shape?

Coffee as well as tea contains caffeine; caffeine is bad for any human being, period. It doesn't matter to me if you are trying to lose weight or gain it or whatever, a large intake of caffeine can affect many different functions of the human body, especially metabolism.

How can a personal trainer help a client, with regard to nutrition?

Depending on an individual goal of the client a personal trainer can recommend a better product and times to eat. There are many products that an average person doesn't know about that actually can be very beneficial to the human body, and many personal trainers are trained in nutrition, so we can recommend the right products.

Is it unhealthy to eat a vegetarian or vegan diet that has no meat or dairy?

No. There are a lot of vegetarians who are working out and healthy without any meat or dairy product intake.

Meat is not the only source of protein that our bodies require. You can find protein in beans, grains, etc. Many people don't know that meat and dairy products make our body very acidic, which creates a great environment in your body for bacteria to grow. And that can be the cause of many illnesses.

Once someone begins working out with a personal trainer, what goes on during the sessions?

Warm-up, main personalized workout program, warm-down, stretches. You want to make sure that the workout is done in a proper order which can maximum the benefit for the client and get desirable results. First workout sessions are mostly focused on getting familiar with exercise equipment, technical aspects of a body movement (proper technique is essential), proper breathing and recovery time. Later on it is much easier to keep the workout session in a right tempo, since a client knows the routine.

How long should a personal training session last?

It depends on a goals of the client. On average 1-1.5 hours. It is absolutely unnecessary to have a long workout as the client has to stay focused, on target and hydrated. Many people go to a local gym to socialize rather than workout; that is why having a personal trainer is essential for most people.

How much will it cost to hire a personal trainer?

The cost to hire a personal trainer may vary from city to city. California might be slightly more expansive than Ohio for example. I charge $70 per session. The more sessions my client buys the cheaper it is. Like 8 sessions for $400.

Is it better to work out for a long period of time at a low intensity or a short period of time at a high intensity?

If you are working out to build a stamina and endurance then a long period at a low intensity is better. If you are working on burning calories a short period at a high intensity would be required. Also, if you are working on building muscles (hypertrophy) then the workout has to be done at a steady pace with up to 2 minute breaks between the repetitions.

How do people get rid of loose skin after weight loss?

The fastest way is plastic surgery. The smartest way is to lose weight slowly (gradually) without shocking changes to your body, so your body parts: bones, skin, joints, etc. have time to adjust naturally to changes.

Change in diet by adding vitamins, minerals or essential oils might smooth the recovery.

How do people measure their heart rate?

You will need find your maximum heart rate (MHR) by subtracting your age from 220, then multiple (MHR) by 0.60 - lower end of the target heart rate zone, then multiply (MHR) by 0.90 - upper end of the target heart rate zone. You want to stay between these numbers during your workout.

Why is it that, no matter how much cardio some people do, they still can't lose weight?

It has to do with many factors, but the formula to lose weight is simple: Incoming calories VS outgoing calories. Incoming calories always have to be lower than the outgoing calories. Many people think that by working out more they don't have to watch what and how much they eat; unfortunately they do. There are many programs available to count your calories. I do recommend eating more alkaline products and consuming protein separately from carbohydrates, so your body doesn't get too toxic and acidic. So far my clients have had great results.

Do men lose weight faster than women?

Not necessarily. Men do build muscles much better and faster than women, thanks to higher testosterone levels in men's bodies. If men or women are following the same formula: Incoming calories (food) VS outgoing calories (exercise), then it shouldn't matter. The main reason for women losing weight slower could be a disbalance in a hormone level in her body. Usually, it changes with age after age 50+ or if they take some sort of medicine. But it is also a possibility that they have an illness and consulting a doctor is recommended.

Is there an ideal time of day to work out?

It totally depends on the client's biorhythms. Many people are getting great results by working out in the morning, but many get great results by doing it in evening. It any case it is recommended to workout 2-3 hours before bed time. My client's busy schedules change all the time, so we have to find a good time so they are not too tired and have enough energy left over for a great workout.

Columbus Dance Centre

1000-B Morrison Rd

Gahanna, OH 43230

614-759-0502

www.columbusdancecentre.com

8 ANDREW JOHNSTON

Triumph Training

St. Petersburg, FL

President/Owner

Andrew founded Triumph Training in 2000, turning his athletic experience and insatiable appetite for knowledge into a successful training business. Not content with having obtained his Certified Strength and Conditioning Specialist degree, arguably the most respected credential in the fitness industry, Andrew became the first Corrective Holistic Exercise Kinesiologist in the state of Georgia in 2001. His passion for the body and its limitless potential has since grown only stronger with Men's Journal naming him one of the Best Trainers in the U.S. in 2005 and again in 2006. Perfecting what he preaches to his clientele as well as various audiences throughout the Southeast, in 2006 Andrew became the first Leukemia Survivor to qualify for and finish the Hawaii Ironman World Championships. The award-winning documentary Living is Winning captures the events leading up to that race and takes the audience deep into the life of an aspiring triathlete. Now he takes his knowledge as a Holistic Lifestyle Coach and CHEK practitioner to guide people in their pursuit of wellness, ultimately helping them to realize that the only limitations they truly have are the ones they set for themselves.

If someone eats very healthy, and they have an active lifestyle, do they still need to work out? Why or why not?

One should only workout when they are healthy enough for an exercise program. Exercise is a stress. And if you stress a system which is already in the red, you end up breaking that system. Thus, eating healthy and maintaining an active lifestyle are essential prerequisites before undertaking an exercise program. Then, the exercise chosen should reflect both what the person needs and what the person wants to do. This last point is critical: in an experiment with rats, researchers found that when they let a rat run on a wheel at the rat's discretion, all health markers improved. However, when the rat was forced to run, those same health markers declined.

Do minors typically need to get the permission of an adult or guardian, if they want to work with a personal trainer? If so, how does this work?

Yes--I require anyone below the age of 18 to have permission from a parent/guardian. This is included in my typical intake forms.

Why do some people lift heavy weights while other people lift lighter amounts of weights?

There are various reasons to lift at various intensities. But oftentimes, misconceptions are what leads a person to choose a particular weight. The idea that weight training makes a person big or bulky is a fallacy--one which motivates many women to stick to light weights. However, muscle hypertrophy occurs primarily at an intensity (i.e. weight) which allows the lifter to perform between 8 and 12 repetitions. Thus, lifting a weight which can be lifted 20 times or more is not intense enough to stimulate much growth. Muscular endurance is what is being trained at higher rep ranges. And while challenging, this is considered high density training, not high intensity training. A weight which can only be lifted say 4 times or less will also not stimulate much growth as the volume necessary to illicit the muscle to get bigger. This is considered maximum strength or power work (depending on the tempo used) and will not result in a large increase in muscle mass. And while both lifting scenarios have their particular effects on the body, muscular size is not a common characteristic of either one.

Do personal trainers normally work with clients who are only free on weekends or during off-hours? What's typical in terms of when personal trainers are available?

I work one-on-one with clients only Monday-Friday and only between the hours of 7 a.m. and 6 p.m. Those parameters help to maintain marital bliss and allow me to have time to pursue goals outside of my profession. Most trainers will find clients who prefer early a.m. or later p.m. slots as work limits when they can be with a trainer. However, the hours in which a trainer will typically work is typically based on the trainer's discretion.

If someone has back problems, or other physical limitations, how can they lift weights safely, without getting hurt?

A person with back pain or any orthopedic limitation can strength train safely if the program being followed is the right one. The first meeting or two with me is not what some might expect. I take my clients through an extensive session (typically lasting a total of 3hrs) which entail postural analysis, testing of core function, movement screens to determine strengths/weaknesses/areas of concern, length tension relationships, neurological screening, and more.

With this information, design a workout to address any physiological issue (known or unknown) which may preclude the client from reaching his/her athletic potential/fitness goal. Without this knowledge, one is not only wasting their time; they're likely going down the path of injury as well. In other words, if you're not assessing, you're guessing. Though most trainers don't realize this, exercise is powerful medicine and needs to be prescribed accordingly. That's what I do.

What is the typical way to pay a personal trainer? Weekly? Monthly? At each session?

Many trainers prefer to sell packages, often discounting their services according to how many sessions are purchased. I don't work that way. I place a value on my time which doesn't change according to how often a person sees me. In fact, my business model is not a revolving door one. I'm a success when clients walk through my door because they want to see me, not because they have to see me. I realize that my clients all have the potential to be self-sufficient and achieve almost anything they can imagine. In fact, I believe in them more than they believe in themselves sometimes. So I try to "teach them how to fish" rather than "giving them a fish". Otherwise, I'm just an expensive babysitter in a co-dependent relationship--and that's not healthy for either of us.

When is a spotter needed for exercises?

A spotter is needed for exercise whenever the strength or proficiency of the exerciser is in question in regards to a particular movement. Except in cases of learning a new exercise or maximum strength training, the need for a spotter brings into question the appropriateness of a particular movement for that person.

How does someone tone up in specific "problem areas"?

There is no such thing as "spot" reduction. That's a common fallacy. A tendency to gain weight in a certain area is dependent on genetics and nutrition/lifestyle. Thus, countering unwanted weight gain in a particular area is often best addressed by optimizing how a person thinks, breathes, drinks, eats, and sleeps.

Is it true that too much cardio can be unhealthy?

The only time our ancestors ever did "cardio" was when they were either running for their lives or fighting for their lives. Thus, cardio as is typically performed (i.e. abused) triggers the sympathetic nervous system (SNS). In contrast to the parasympathetic nervous system (PNS), the SNS triggers the release of stress hormones like cortisol and adrenalin and puts the body in a catabolic state, decreasing muscle mass, inhibiting immunity, and a host of other detrimental effects. Additionally, when the SNS is stimulated, the PNS is proportionally inhibited. Since digestion and repair are key aspects of the PNS, these critical processes don't occur. The stressors of everyday life (work, relationships, dehydration, poor food choices, lack of sleep, etc.) will often cause a person to be in SNS dominant mode. Therefore, pushing a person further into a state of SNS dominance is something which should be avoided. Cardio can be performed safely if used judiciously and at appropriate intensities/frequencies for a particular person. Commonly, however, people aren't healthy enough for the demands cardio, as typically carried, out put on the body.

What are the benefits of hiring a personal trainer over just buying some DVDs that feature personal trainers?

One man's medicine is another man's poison. A one-size-fits-all approach to exercise never works for everyone and rarely works for anyone. "Personal" is in the word personal trainer for a reason. Unfortunately, the state of personal training is in such a state that this idea has largely been forgotten.

Is it a good idea to walk or run with weights? Will this produce results more quickly?
Vladimir Janda says it takes as little as 3 days to change gait. Walking or running with weights is a recipe for dysfunction as the cumulative effect of walking/running with compensatory motions to which the body has not adequately adapted will eventually result in injury.

How soon, after someone starts a diet and exercise program, should they start to see results, to know if their diet and exercise program is working?

It's not just about how you look in the mirror. While you cannot be fat and healthy, you can easily be skinny and unhealthy. So seeing results should be second to feeling results. When on the right program, a person should feel his/her level of vitality increasing, and their performance as well as their body will ultimately reflect that.

What are some of the most common misconceptions that people have about hiring a personal trainer?

Hiring a personal trainer is where it ends. But you still have to put in the effort. And that work begins by doing the research and finding a trainer who has more than a simple certification which is worth less than the paper on which it's printed.

What are some of the most common myths about nutrition?

That just about anything the USDA says is good for you is actually healthy. They have it all wrong, and their recommendations are motivated more by money and the lobby of certain special interest groups like the grain lobby or the chemical industry. Just look around at the state of health is the U.S. today. 2/3 of us are overweight. 1/2 of us will develop cancer. Adult onset diabetes had to be renamed Type 2 diabetes due to its prevalence in children. For the first time in recorded history, life expectancy went down in the country.

Quite frankly, your great grandparents knew more about health and nutrition than the government does today.

What are some of the biggest mistakes that people make when they start an exercise program?

Too much too soon. It's about training, not draining. Do don't expect overnight results. Quick typically means temporary. More importantly, it also means unhealthy. Slow and steady wins this race. It's a lifestyle--not a weekstyle! So find something which works for you and build health and happiness on a foundation of common sense and consistency.

Andrew Johnston

Triumph Training

www.triumphtraining.com
404/431-2287

Author of Holistic Strength Training for Triathlon, Andrew is a former professional cyclist, the first leukemia survivor to qualify for and finish the Hawaii Ironman World Championships, the creator of Daily Tips for Holistic Health for I-Phones, and twice voted One of the Top Trainers in America by Men's Health.

9 MICHAEL BLAUNER

Personal Fitness by Michael Blauner
Ridgewood, NJ
Owner

From celebrities and titans of wall street, to your neighbor on Main street. Since 1986 Michael Blauner has been one of New Jersey's leading personal trainers.

His motivational skills and training techniques have helped so many achieve and maintain their fitness goals. no matter what level of fitness, Michael is adept at training absolute beginners as well as competitive athletes. Michael welcomes all. The program is structured around your busy schedule and tailored to suit your physical capabilities and needs.

The new fad seems to be "buying organic". Is there any validity to eating organic food over non-organic food? What are the benefits and/or things to be aware of?

I don't think I would call buying organic a fad at this point. Many of the things I see being sold on the infomercials are much more of a fad! There is a very deep divide over the necessity of buying organic. Personally I feel that it is overrated. I am confident with our regulations over non organic food and that they are completely safe and healthy. Granted, not having chemicals involved in the growth of food products is a very good thing , however; when it comes to fruits and vegetables ,if you are concerned , you can spend a little time cleaning them thoroughly to remove any residual chemicals. The added cost of these foods just doesn't add up in my opinion.

Should people wait until they're not sore from their previous workout to start working out again?

I am not a believer in pushing people to the point of overdoing it. Training should leave people feeling good. It should be a gradual build up that will lead to a healthy fit body. A little feeling of soreness is a nice way to remind yourself that you worked out, but anything beyond that is your body telling you that you are at risk of injury. So if you need to wait to work out because you are too sore... you should reconsider what you are doing in the first place.

If someone reaches their fitness goals, should they still continue to work with a personal trainer?

Well, of course, my opinion is that everyone needs a personal trainer! If you used a trainer to reach your goals and are considering not using said trainer anymore you must realize that, whatever you have done to get to your current fitness level is exactly what you must continue to do to maintain this level. If you can motivate and push yourself on a regular basis then great. If not, and you don't want the continued expense, you might want to cut back and use your trainer for maintenance. For instance, work with your trainer once a week for real motivation and train on your own two other times a week. This will keep your routine fresh and you will definitely be more apt to stay the course!

When people first start exercising, why do they sometimes gain weight initially?

Often people gain weight when they first start working out for a couple of reasons; one reason is that as your muscles are being used in ways that they haven't experienced in a while , they will look to retain water as part of the process of development, and this is a good , healthy thing. This retention of water can cause a gain in weight. The muscles will draw water within making them more dense [heavier] and become fit and strong. On the other hand exercise stimulates your appetite. As you are burning more calories by exercising your newly elevated metabolism will tell your body to replace the calories it burned and then some! Look at the metabolic functions as a furnace, as you work harder the furnace looks to be fed energy. Avoid high calorie junk food and foods loaded with processed sugars. Feed it healthy good quality food and all should be OK!

If someone has a heart condition, can they still workout?

In so many cases if people exercised in the first place they wouldn't have a heart condition. Most all cardiologists recognize this. As a result of that they will commonly prescribe exercise, in a controlled environment, to rehab cardio patients. So what could have been the prevention also becomes the cure! It is highly recommended that if you have cardiovascular disease you need to consult your doctor before embarking on any exercise program. Exercise is good for everything.

If someone has a job where they don't move around a lot, what can they do to increase their activity during the day, when they're not working out?

I always tell my clients who have office jobs that the best thing they can do during the day is to stand up. This act alone keeps the body strong and more in line than if you were just sitting all day. You keep your back muscles erect and your stomach in check. The tendency to slump forward has terrible long term effects on the body. Of course I would always recommend that people should do a set of pushups any chance they get as well as a set of deep knee bends/squats. These are things that stimulate your metabolism and keep you strong. So close the office door and do 10 pushups!

Is it safe for pregnant women to work out?

If a woman is already in shape and has been working out all along then with some doctor recommended changes to her program she can certainly continue to exercise. However, it is not wise to be out of shape and then to begin a program when you find out you are pregnant. So here the answer is; always try to stay in shape and then this will not be a concern.

If someone prefers to work out without a personal trainer, can a trainer still help them get started? How would this work?

If someone prefers to work out on their own and finds it productive... then great! In order to get started on the right foot there are many trainers that would be happy to help and you could hire them on a as needed basis. If only there were more people who have the drive to do so on a regular basis then this country wouldn't be facing ever increasing rates of obesity.

Can someone use a personal trainer to help them rehabilitate from a sports injury? How would this be handled?

Physical therapy is best for most people coming off of an injury. Personal training can help get you and keep you in shape. And if you are training correctly then the chance of injury is greatly reduced. That is about as far as a trainer should claim that they can do for healing injuries. An injury and subsequent rehab should be handled by the professionals who deal with such issues.

When it comes to nutrition, it seems that few experts can agree on what is a healthy diet and what is not. How can people know which advice to take, with all of the contradictory information out there?

Actually I don't think there is too much contrary advice on what is healthy nutrition and what isn't. Everyone at this point knows. Granted, you have debates between vegetarians and meat eaters, organic and non-organic etc... however if you look at the big picture what these food conscious people all agree on is eat as many unprocessed whole foods as possible, don't overeat, and exercise on a regular basis.

Is it a good idea to eat any specific foods immediately before or after exercising?

You can never drink enough water before, during and after your workout. I always tell clients to consume some form of carbohydrate before their workout, for energy [orange juice is very effective] and try to eat some protein shortly thereafter for the benefits of muscular development.

Should people with low blood sugar do anything differently before, during, or after a workout?

I myself often feel the negative effects of low blood sugar, so here as previously mentioned I highly recommend keeping orange juice or something similar to it handy. If you go to a sporting goods store ask for the pre-packed instant gels that runners use while training; they are very useful as well. The benefits are instant and will allow you to continue with your workout in the way you want.

Is it true that it's bad to eat too much fruit because of all of the sugar it contains?

I have never seen anyone gain weight from eating too much fruit!! It's quite the opposite; they gain weight because they don't eat fruit.

What precautions should seniors take into consideration, when starting a new exercise program?

Like almost everyone else seniors should consult with their physician before embarking on an exercise program. Find something you enjoy which will keep you interested and take it slow in the beginning. Everyone should build gradually and because there is a slightly higher risk of injury in the senior population they should take extra care. But by all means the benefits and gains in strength has been seen to be tremendous amongst seniors who newly embark on a safe guided program.

What are some simple things that people can do, in their day to day routine, besides working out, to see results faster?

I am all about simplicity. So here are a few things people can do to see great results without consuming their life. Drink a lot of water. Walk a mile as often as you can. Eat a lot of fruits and vegetables. Don't smoke. Keep alcohol intake limited. Do a set of pushups every day. Take the necessary vitamins. Limit your red meat consumption. Read a book a month. Try to laugh as often as possible. And try not to let the little things bother you!

I can be contacted through my website:

michaelblauner.com
phone 201-665-0591

CONCLUSION

Congratulations on making it to the end of this book! We hope that you realize and appreciate the immense level of real world knowledge that you've just acquired. The one thing you may be feeling, at this point, is a bit of "information overload", due to the many tips, pieces of advice, and strategies that are jammed into this book. If you are feeling a bit overwhelmed from everything you've just learned, allow us to offer you one final piece of advice: Take a day to let your brain absorb all of the information you just learned. As they say: "Sleep on it". If you attempt to try and remember and implement everything you just learned, your efforts may tend to be scattered and a bit unorganized. Instead, take a day off from the information. If you do this, you're likely to find that you develop a sense of clarity and a better perspective on the information.

Once you've taken a day to allow yourself to re-focus in this way, we encourage you to slowly go back through the book, writing down the actionable information that you intend to implement. Simply reading and understanding the information is not enough. By writing down the information that you plan on implementing, it will allow you to put a clear plan of action into place for yourself.

As you go through the information, don't worry about the order in which you write things down. The first thing to do is to just get the information down on paper. There are many great strategies and tips within this book, but the goal here is for you to extract the exact advice that you will be taking action on. Don't worry if you are unsure about whether or not you will be taking immediate action on certain advice. Just write down everything that you may possibly take action on.

Once you've compiled this list of action steps and "maybe action steps", begin to prioritize this list. In other words, re-write the list with the actions that you know you're going to take at the top of the list and the action items that you may not take action on towards the bottom of the list. By organizing your list in this way, you will be able to build a practical, useable to-do list, from the information you learned in this book. Once you've done this, you will be in an excellent position to start taking focused steps, with clarity and purpose.

As we mentioned at the beginning of this book, most peddlers of fitness products and information hope that you keep buying their stuff. In keeping with the rebellious nature of this book, we encourage you to stop buying more fitness stuff and start implementing what you just learned in this book! Just as we have shared interviews with real world experts who actually do what they talk about in this book, it is our hope that you, as the reader, will take real world action on the information you've learned here.

Wishing you all the best in your action-taking, fitness and nutrition endeavors!

www.ingramcontent.com/pod-product-compliance
Lightning Source LLC
Chambersburg PA
CBHW072338290526
45794CB00002B/929